WALL PILATES FOR MEN OVER 50

50+ Exercises For Beginners And Seniors To Enhance Mobility, Strength And Balance

Randy T. Luca

Copyright 2023, Randy T. Lucas

All rights reserved. No part of this publication may be reproduced, stored in a retrieval system, or transmitted, in any form or by any means, electronic, mechanical, photocopying, recording, or otherwise, without the prior written permission of the author, except in the case of brief quotations embodied in critical reviews and certain other noncommercial uses permitted by copyright law.

Table of contents

INTRODUCTION:

Mark was in his late 50s, feeling the gradual effects of aging taking a toll on his body. As a man who always valued an active lifestyle, he found himself searching for a way to maintain his fitness while addressing the specific needs of his age group. That's when he discovered Wall Pilates.

Through consistent practice, Mark experienced a transformation. His posture improved, his core strengthened, and he regained flexibility he hadn't felt in years. Wall Pilates became more than just a workout routine; it became a rejuvenating experience that empowered him to embrace life with renewed vigor.

Welcome to "Wall Pilates for Men Over 50," a comprehensive guide designed to introduce you to the transformative power of Pilates exercises using a wall as your ally. In this guide, we delve into the unique benefits that Wall Pilates offers specifically tailored to the needs of men navigating the journey of aging.

As men enter their 50s and beyond, maintaining fitness becomes not only essential but also a key factor in sustaining a high quality of life. Wall Pilates, a derivative of traditional Pilates exercises, incorporates the stability and support of a wall, making it an ideal practice for men in this age group. It offers a low-impact yet highly effective way to build strength, enhance flexibility, and improve overall well-being.

In this guide, you'll discover a curated collection of exercises, techniques, and strategies designed to help you navigate the world of Wall Pilates confidently. Whether you're new to Pilates or a seasoned practitioner, the exercises presented here cater specifically to the needs and challenges commonly faced by men over 50.

The journey of exploring Wall Pilates is not just about physical exercise; it's about finding balance, enhancing mobility, and nurturing a deeper connection between mind and body. As you embark on this journey, remember that consistency and dedication will be your allies in reaping the countless benefits that Wall Pilates has to offer.

So, let's step closer to vitality, strength, and a renewed sense of well-being through the enriching practice of Wall Pilates.

CHAPTER 1

Understanding Wall Pilates for Men Over 50

What is Pilates?

Pilates is a comprehensive and mindful exercise system that focuses on strengthening the body, improving flexibility, and enhancing overall well-being. Developed by Joseph Pilates in the early 20th century, this method was initially called "Contrology" and was designed to create a harmonious connection between the body and mind.

At its core, Pilates emphasizes precise and controlled movements, breathing techniques, and proper body alignment. The exercises are designed to engage the deep stabilizing muscles of the core, including the abdominals, back muscles, pelvic floor, and muscles supporting the spine. This focus on the core provides a strong foundation for all movements while promoting better posture and spinal alignment.

Pilate's exercises can be performed on a mat using body weight or with specialized equipment such as the Reformer, Cadillac, or Wunda Chair, which utilize springs and resistance to add challenge and variety to workouts. These exercises are adaptable and can be modified to accommodate various fitness levels, making Pilates suitable for beginners as well as athletes and individuals recovering from injuries.

The benefits of Pilates are extensive. It helps in building long, lean muscles without adding bulk, improving flexibility, and enhancing muscular endurance. Moreover, Pilates aids in developing body awareness, balance, and coordination. It is renowned for its ability to alleviate back pain, strengthen the core, and rehabilitate injuries, especially related to the spine and joints.

One of the distinguishing features of Pilates is its emphasis on the mind-body connection. Practitioners are encouraged to focus on breathing patterns, concentration, and precision of movements during exercises. This holistic approach not only contributes to physical fitness but also promotes relaxation, stress reduction, and mental clarity.

Pilates is widely embraced by people of all ages and fitness levels, from athletes looking to enhance performance to individuals seeking a gentle yet effective form of exercise. Its adaptability, focus on core strength, and emphasis on mindful movement make Pilates a versatile and beneficial practice for achieving overall wellness and a healthier lifestyle.

Benefits of Pilates for men over 50

1. Improved Posture: Pilates helps strengthen core muscles, promoting better posture, reducing back pain, and enhancing overall spinal alignment, crucial for combating the effects of aging on posture.

2. Enhanced Flexibility: The controlled movements and stretches in Pilates exercises contribute to increased flexibility, aiding in maintaining mobility and preventing muscle stiffness often experienced with age.

3. Core Strength: Pilates targets the deep core muscles, providing stability and strength essential for maintaining balance and preventing injuries, particularly beneficial as individual's age.

4. Muscle Tone and Strength: Pilates focuses on full-body workouts, helping men over 50 build lean muscle mass, improve muscular endurance, and regain strength without putting excessive strain on joints.

5. Balance and Coordination: As men age, balance and coordination tend to decline. Pilate's exercises challenge these aspects, enhancing stability and coordination through controlled movements and balance-focused exercises.

6. Joint Health and Flexibility: Gentle yet effective, Pilates promotes joint mobility and flexibility, which can alleviate stiffness and reduce the risk of joint-related issues often associated with aging.

7. Stress Reduction and Mental Well-being: The mindful aspect of Pilates, combined with its emphasis on breathing techniques, aids in stress reduction, promotes relaxation, and supports mental clarity and focus.

8. Injury Prevention: By strengthening muscles and improving flexibility, Pilates lowers the risk of injury, particularly for men over 50 who may be more susceptible to muscle strains or joint injuries.

9. Improved Circulation: Through controlled movements and enhanced breathing, Pilates exercises facilitate better blood circulation, benefiting cardiovascular health and overall well-being.

10. Tailored to Individual Needs: Pilates can be modified to accommodate various fitness levels and specific health concerns, making it an adaptable practice for men over 50 with different abilities and conditions.

These benefits collectively make Pilates an excellent choice for men over 50 seeking to maintain or enhance their physical fitness, flexibility, and overall well-being as they navigate the aging process.

Why Use a Wall for Pilates Exercises?

1. Stability and Support: The wall provides a stable surface for support and balance, especially beneficial for beginners or those with balance issues. It allows individuals to focus on proper form and technique without worrying about maintaining balance, reducing the risk of injury.

2. Alignment Assistance: Utilizing a wall helps in maintaining proper body alignment during exercises. It acts as a visual and tactile guide, enabling practitioners to align their posture correctly, promoting better spinal alignment and reducing strain on the back and neck.

3. Increased Intensity and Resistance: By pressing against the wall during certain exercises, individuals can create added resistance, intensifying the workout. This added resistance challenges muscles further, enhancing strength and toning.

4. Versatility in Exercise Variation: The wall offers versatility, allowing for a wider range of exercise variations and modifications. It enables modifications to accommodate different fitness levels, making Pilates accessible and adaptable for individuals with varying abilities.

5. Enhanced Stretching and Range of Motion: The wall serves as a tool for deeper stretching and increased range of motion. It aids in achieving better stretches for various muscle groups, promoting flexibility and aiding in muscle recovery after workouts.

Overall, incorporating a wall into Pilates exercises not only adds stability and support but also allows for greater versatility, improved alignment, enhanced resistance, and increased stretching benefits. This integration contributes significantly to a more comprehensive and effective Pilates workout regimen.

CHAPTER 2

Basic Wall Pilates Exercises

Breathing Techniques in Pilates:

1. Diaphragmatic Breathing Exercise:

- Stand or sit comfortably with your spine straight, shoulders relaxed.

- Place one hand on your chest and the other on your abdomen.

- Inhale deeply through your nose, feeling your abdomen expand as you breathe in.

- Exhale slowly through pursed lips, feeling your abdomen gently contract.

- Focus on breathing deeply into your diaphragm, allowing your chest to remain relatively still.

2. Rib Cage Expansion Breathing:

- Sit or stand tall, placing your hands on the sides of your rib cage.

- Inhale deeply through your nose, expanding your rib cage outward to the sides.

- Exhale slowly through your mouth, feeling your ribs gently contract.

- Concentrate on expanding the sides of your rib cage while maintaining a relaxed posture.

3. Segmental Breathing Exercise:

- Lie on your back with knees bent and feet flat on the floor.

- Place one hand on your chest and the other on your abdomen.

- Inhale deeply, directing the breath sequentially into different sections of your lungs (lower, middle, upper).

- Exhale slowly, focusing on emptying the lungs in reverse order (upper, middle, lower).

Warm-Up Exercises:

1. Neck Rolls:

- Stand tall or sit comfortably with your spine straight.

- Gently drop your chin to your chest and roll your head to the right, then slowly circle it around to the left, completing a full rotation.

- Reverse the direction and repeat for several rotations, keeping movements slow and controlled.

2. Arm Circles:

- Stand with feet hip-width apart and arms extended straight out to the sides at shoulder height.

- Begin making small circles with your arms, gradually increasing the size of the circles.

- Reverse the direction after several repetitions, maintaining controlled and smooth movements.

3. Leg Swings:

- Stand facing the wall with one hand placed lightly on it for balance.

- Swing one leg forward and backward in a controlled manner, maintaining a straight leg and flexing the foot.

- Switch to the other leg and repeat the swinging motion, focusing on increasing the range of motion gradually.

Posture Alignment against the Wall:

1. Wall Standing Posture Check:

- Stand with your back against a wall, heels slightly away, and feet hip-width apart.
- Ensure your head, shoulder blades, and hips are in contact with the wall.
- Gently press the small of your back against the wall, maintaining a natural curve in your spine.
- Hold this position for 30 seconds to 1 minute, focusing on alignment and breathing.

2. Wall Angel Exercise:

- Stand with your back against the wall and arms bent at a 90-degree angle, palms facing forward.

- Slowly slide your arms up the wall while keeping contact with your elbows, wrists, and back.

- Return to the starting position, ensuring your back maintains contact with the wall throughout the movement.

3. Wall Spine Stretch:

- Stand against the wall with your feet slightly away from it.

- Slowly slide down the wall, bending your knees and rolling your spine onto the wall, until you reach a comfortable squat position.

- Hold for a few seconds, then return to standing by pushing through your heels and straightening your legs.

Wall Squats and Modifications:

1. Basic Wall Squat:

- Stand with your back against the wall and feet shoulder-width apart.
- Bend your knees and slide slowly down the wall until your thighs are parallel to the floor.
- Hold this position for a few seconds, then push through your heels to return to the starting position.

2. One-Leg Wall Squat:

- Similar to the basic wall squat, but lift one foot slightly off the ground, extending it in front of you.
- Perform the wall squat movement using only one leg, ensuring the other leg remains lifted throughout the exercise.
- Alternate between legs for a balanced workout.

3. Ball Squeeze Wall Squat:

- Place a small exercise ball between your lower back and the wall.

- Perform the wall squat exercise while maintaining pressure against the ball throughout the movement, engaging core muscles for added stability.

CHAPTER 3

Intermediate Wall Pilates Exercises

Wall Roll-Downs and Spinal Mobility:

1. Standing Wall Roll-Downs:

- Place your feet hip-width apart and lean your back against the wall.

- Begin by gently tucking your chin to your chest and slowly roll down through the spine, segment by segment, as if peeling away from the wall.

- Keep knees slightly bent as you articulate down, aiming to touch the floor or go as far as comfortable.

- Roll back up to the starting position, one vertebra at a time, returning to standing against the wall.

2. Wall Articulation with Arm Reach:

- Stand facing the wall, arms extended forward at shoulder height, palms pressing against the wall.

- Slowly articulate the spine, rolling down as before, while simultaneously reaching your arms higher along the wall.

- Hold the forward bend position briefly, then articulate the spine back up while lowering the arms to shoulder height.

3. Pelvic Tilt against the Wall:

- Place your feet hip-width apart and lean your back against the wall, and knees slightly bent.

- Gently press your lower back into the wall, engaging your abdominal muscles.

- Slowly tilt your pelvis up and down, maintaining contact with the wall, to enhance pelvic mobility and spinal awareness.

Leg Raises and Abdominal Strengthening:

1. Single Leg Raises against the Wall:

- Place your hands beneath your hips for support while lying on your back with your legs extended against the wall.

- Lift one leg vertically towards the ceiling while keeping the other leg against the wall.

- Lower the raised leg back down and switch to the other leg, alternating leg raises while engaging the core.

2. Wall Scissor Kicks:

- Place your hands beneath your hips for support while lying on your back with your legs extended against the wall.

- Lift both legs slightly off the wall, then scissor them back and forth, crossing one leg over the other and alternating positions.

3. Leg Circles against the Wall:

- Place your hands beneath your hips for support while lying on your back with your legs extended against the wall.

- Keeping one leg against the wall, circle the other leg in a controlled motion, drawing circles on the wall in both clockwise and counterclockwise directions.

Wall Planks and Variations:

1. Forearm Wall Plank:

- Assume a plank position with forearms resting against the wall, elbows directly under shoulders, and body in a straight line from head to heels.
- Hold this position, engaging core muscles and keeping the back flat, aiming for a stable and controlled posture.

2. High Wall Plank with Shoulder Taps:

- Assume a plank position with hands against the wall, arms fully extended, and body straight from head to heels.
- While maintaining a stable plank, alternately tap your shoulders with your hands, focusing on minimizing body sway.

3. Wall Side Plank:

- Lie on your side with feet stacked against the wall and forearm supporting your upper body.

- Lift your hips off the floor, forming a straight line from head to heels, engaging core muscles, and holding the side plank position. Repeat on both sides.

Chest Openers and Shoulder Mobility:

1. Wall Chest Opener Stretch:

- Stand perpendicular to the wall with one arm extended and resting against it at shoulder height.

- Gently rotate away from the wall, opening the chest and feeling a stretch across the front of the shoulder and chest.

- Hold the stretch, then switch sides and repeat.

2. Wall Shoulder Blade Squeeze:

- Stand against the wall with arms bent at 90 degrees and elbows at shoulder height.

- Squeeze your shoulder blades together, pressing them against the wall, while maintaining the arm position.

- Hold for a few seconds, then release and repeat, focusing on proper shoulder blade engagement.

3. Wall Arm Circles for Shoulder Mobility:

- Stand facing the wall with arms extended at shoulder height and palms pressed against the wall.

- Begin making small circles with your arms on the wall, gradually increasing the size of the circles while maintaining contact with the wall.

- Reverse the direction after several repetitions, focusing on smooth and controlled movements to enhance shoulder mobility.

CHAPTER 4

Advanced Wall Pilates Exercises

Wall Push-Ups and Variations:

1. Traditional Wall Push-Up:

- Stand facing the wall, arms extended at shoulder height and palms against the wall.

- Bend your elbows to bring your chest closer to the wall, then push yourself back to the starting position.

- Perform push-ups with controlled movements, focusing on engaging the chest, shoulders, and triceps.

2. Decline Wall Push-Ups:

- Assume a plank position with feet elevated against the wall and hands on the floor slightly wider than shoulder-width apart.

- Perform push-ups by lowering your chest towards the ground, maintaining a straight line from head to heels.

3. One-Arm Wall Push-Up:

- Stand facing the wall and place one hand against the wall at shoulder height.

- Perform push-ups using only one arm, maintaining stability and balance while engaging the chest and arm muscles.

Single Leg Wall Squats and Balance Work:

1. Single Leg Wall Squat with Reach:

- Stand on one leg facing the wall, with the other leg extended forward.

- Perform a single leg wall squat, lowering yourself toward the wall while reaching the opposite hand towards the wall.

- Focus on balance, control, and maintaining stability throughout the movement.

2. Single Leg Wall Squat with Rotation:

- Stand on one leg facing the wall, with the other leg extended forward.

- Perform a single leg wall squat while twisting your torso and reaching the opposite hand across your body towards the wall.

- Engage core muscles to maintain balance and control.

3. Single Leg Wall Squat with Knee Drive:

- Stand on one leg facing the wall, with the other leg extended forward.

- Perform a single leg wall squat, then drive the knee of the extended leg up towards your chest while maintaining balance and control.

- Return to the starting position and repeat, focusing on stability and core engagement.

Wall-Assisted Inversions for Flexibility:

1. Wall Supported Headstand Preparation:

- Kneel facing away from the wall, interlace fingers and place forearms on the floor, creating a triangle base with your head inside.
- Lift hips toward the ceiling, walk feet in towards your body, and gently place one foot, then the other, against the wall.
- Gradually shift weight onto the forearms, aiming for a supported headstand position, ensuring stability and safety.

2. Wall-Assisted Shoulder Stand:

- Lie on your back close to the wall, lift legs towards the ceiling, and use the wall for support by placing hands on the lower back.

- Gradually walk feet up the wall, aiming to create a vertical line with your body, allowing the wall to support the legs in a shoulder stand position.

3. Wall-Supported Forward Fold:

- Stand facing the wall with feet hip-width apart.

- Fold forward from the hips, reaching hands towards the floor or resting them on the wall for support, allowing the wall to assist in deepening the forward fold.

Integrating Props for Added Challenge:

1. Resistance Band Wall Pull-Aparts:

- Stand facing the wall, holding a resistance band stretched in front of you at shoulder height.
- Pull the band apart by squeezing your shoulder blades together, then return to the starting position.
- For an added challenge, concentrate on keeping the band tight during the entire exercise.

2. Medicine Ball Wall Throws:

- Stand facing the wall holding a medicine ball at chest level.
- Explosively throw the ball against the wall, catch it, and repeat in a controlled manner.
- Engage core muscles and maintain proper form during the throwing motion.

3. BOSU Ball Wall Squats:

- Place a BOSU ball against the wall, flat side facing out.

- Stand with your back against the BOSU ball and perform wall squats, utilizing the instability of the BOSU for added challenge in balance and muscle engagement.

These exercises represent advanced variations of Wall Pilates, incorporating elements such as single-leg work, inversions, advanced push-up variations, and the use of props to intensify the challenge and effectiveness of the workout for men over 50.

CHAPTER 5

Targeted Focus Areas

Core Strengthening Techniques:

1. Wall Plank with Knee Tucks:

- Put your feet up on the wall and your hands on the floor to form a plank posture.

- Engage core muscles and bring knees towards the chest, alternating between legs while maintaining a stable plank position.

- Focus on controlled movements and core engagement throughout.

2. Wall Sit-Ups:

- Lie on your back with legs extended against the wall and hands behind your head.

- Perform sit-ups by lifting your upper body towards your knees, engaging the core muscles while keeping the legs pressed against the wall.

3. Wall Bridge Exercise:

- Lie on your back with knees bent and feet flat against the wall.

- Lift your hips off the ground, forming a straight line from knees to shoulders, engaging the glutes and core.

- Hold the bridge position for a few seconds, then lower back down and repeat, focusing on maintaining a stable bridge.

Flexibility and Range of Motion:

1. Wall-assisted Hamstring Stretch:

- Lie on your back with one leg extended against the wall and the other extended straight up towards the ceiling.
- Use a towel or strap to gently pull the extended leg towards your head, feeling a stretch in the hamstrings and calf muscles.

2. Wall Hip Opener Stretch:

- Lie on your back perpendicular to the wall, with one leg extended up against the wall and the other leg crossed over it.
- Allow gravity to gently open the hips and stretch the outer hip and glute muscles.

3. Wall Chest Opener Stretch Variation:

- Stand facing the wall and place one hand on the wall at shoulder height, fingers pointing backward.

- Gently rotate your body away from the wall, feeling a stretch across the chest and front of the shoulder.

Injury Prevention and Recovery:

1. Wall-supported Calf Raises:

- Stand facing the wall, placing hands lightly against it for support.

- Rise onto your toes, lifting heels off the ground, then slowly lower back down.

- Perform controlled calf raises to strengthen calf muscles and improve ankle stability.

2. Wall-Assisted Quad Stretch:

- Stand facing the wall, holding onto it with one hand for support.
- Bend one knee, bringing your foot towards your glutes, and gently pull the foot towards your body to stretch the front of the thigh (quadriceps).

3. Wall Hamstring Curls:

- Lie on your back with feet against the wall and knees bent at 90 degrees.
- Lift hips off the ground into a bridge position, then slide feet down the wall, extending legs while engaging the hamstrings, and return to the starting position.

These exercises target specific areas of focus such as core strengthening, flexibility improvement, and injury prevention/recovery, tailored to benefit men over 50 in their fitness and well-being journey.

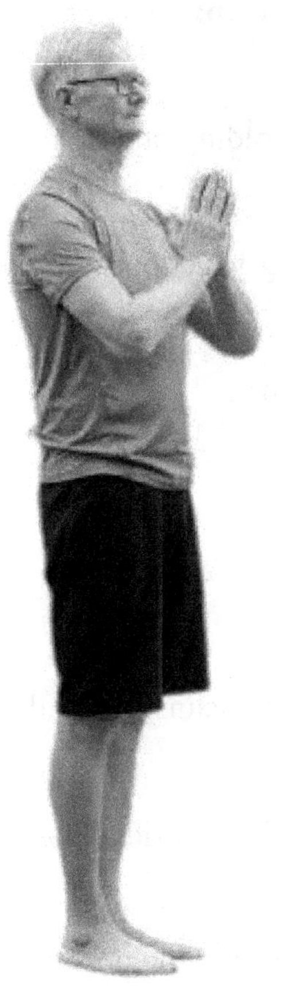

CONCLUSION

In the realm of fitness and holistic well-being, Wall Pilates stands as an invaluable ally for men embarking on the remarkable journey past 50. It's not merely a set of exercises; it's a gateway to transformation, offering a passport to a realm where vitality, strength, and flexibility converge.

As men traverse the terrain of aging, Wall Pilates emerges as a beacon of hope, providing a pathway towards reclaiming physical prowess while nurturing mental equilibrium. The discipline of controlled movements, breathing techniques, and tailored exercises uniquely caters to the needs of those navigating the complexities of age.

What makes Wall Pilates an extraordinary fitness practice for men over 50 is its adaptability. It's not about competition or unattainable goals; it's about personal growth, progress, and embracing one's individual journey to health. The core-strengthening maneuvers, the graceful stretches enhancing flexibility, and the mindful exercises promoting injury prevention are all woven into this tapestry of rejuvenation.

More than the physical gains, Wall Pilates for men over 50 fosters a deeper connection between mind and body. It cultivates resilience, fostering a renewed sense of self-awareness and confidence. With each deliberate breath and each purposeful movement against the wall, a sense of empowerment takes root, allowing these men to stand taller, move more freely, and embrace life's adventures with vigor.

In conclusion, as the curtain falls on this guide, let it mark not an end, but a new beginning. Embrace Wall Pilates as a lifelong companion in the quest for health, vitality, and graceful aging. With dedication, consistency, and an open heart, may the transformative journey through Wall Pilates continue to illuminate the path toward a robust, balanced, and fulfilling life for men over 50.

FITNESS

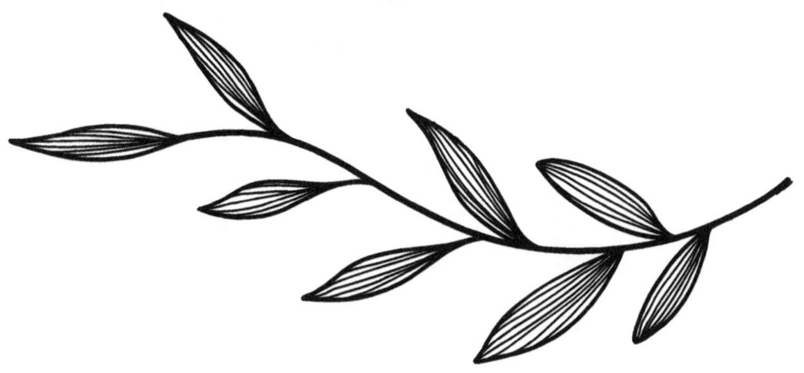

PLANNER

Fitness Planner

NAME: **DATE:**

BREAKFAST

LUNCH

DINNER

SNACK

EXERCISE   SET   REP   NOTES

Fitness Planner

NAME: **DATE:**

BREAKFAST

LUNCH

DINNER

SNACK

EXERCISE

SET	REP	NOTES

Fitness Planner

NAME: **DATE:**

BREAKFAST

LUNCH

DINNER

SNACK

EXERCISE

SET

REP

NOTES

Fitness Planner

NAME: **DATE:**

BREAKFAST

LUNCH

DINNER

SNACK

EXERCISE

SET   REP   NOTES

Fitness Planner

NAME: **DATE:**

BREAKFAST

LUNCH

DINNER

SNACK

EXERCISE

EXERCISE	SET	REP	NOTES

Fitness Planner

NAME:

DATE:

BREAKFAST

LUNCH

DINNER

SNACK

EXERCISE

SET

REP

NOTES

Fitness Planner

NAME: DATE:

BREAKFAST

LUNCH

DINNER

SNACK

EXERCISE   SET   REP   NOTES

Fitness Planner

NAME: **DATE:**

BREAKFAST

LUNCH

DINNER

SNACK

EXERCISE

SET **REP** **NOTES**

Fitness Planner

NAME: **DATE:**

BREAKFAST

LUNCH

DINNER

SNACK

EXERCISE   SET   REP   NOTES

Fitness Planner

NAME: **DATE:**

BREAKFAST

LUNCH

DINNER

SNACK

EXERCISE   SET   REP   NOTES

www.ingramcontent.com/pod-product-compliance
Lightning Source LLC
Chambersburg PA
CBHW061936270726
48660CB00007BA/2784